Super Easy Ve Cookbook

Vegan recipes for everyday meals, learn how to cook easy while having fun. Lose weight fast and begin a new life

Written By

JANE BRACE

Table of Contents

CHOICE CHOCOLATES AND DANDY CANDIES 62

CANDY MAKING BASICS 63

ALLERGY NOTE 81

METRIC CONVERSIONS 92

SORBETS AND ICES

ROSEMARY APPLE SORBET

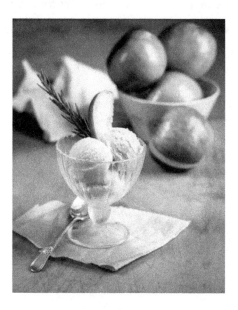

YIELD: 1 QUART

I can't get enough of this sorbet. The apple flavor is really enticing and enhanced elegantly with the addition of rosemary. Be sure to seek out fresh rosemary, rather than dried, as it will absolutely make a difference.

2½ cups apple cider (no sugar added)

⅓ cup sugar

1 sprig fresh rosemary

In a small saucepan over medium heat, combine the apple cider, sugar, and rosemary and cook for about 7 minutes, stirring often, until sugar is dissolved and

11

the rosemary has added a hint of fragrance to the cider. Remove syrup from heat and let cool completely, either in the refrigerator, or at room temperature. Process in ice cream maker according to manufacturer's instructions or by following directions in this book. Once frozen, store in an airtight container in the freezer for up to 2 months.

STRAWBERRIES AND CHAMPAGNE SORBET

YIELD: 1 QUART

I don't actually recommend that you use Champagne to make this delightful sorbet, but you certainly can if you roll hard like that! I prefer Prosecco, for its subtle notes and its more modest price tag.

1 pear, peeled and cubed (about 1 cup)

2 cups strawberries, greens removed

1 cup Prosecco, Spumante, or other sparkling white wine

¾ cup sugar

- In a food processor, pulse together the pear and strawberries until well chopped. In a separate bowl, gradually mix the Prosecco with the sugar and stir gently to dissolve. Let rest for about 5 minutes and then stir gently again. Drizzle about ½ cup of the Prosecco mixture into the food processor and blend until quite smooth, for about 1 minute, scraping down the bowl as needed.

- Add in the rest of the Prosecco mixture and blend until very well combined. Transfer to the bowl of an ice cream maker and process according to manufacturer's instructions or by following directions on <u>in this book</u>.

- Store in an airtight container for up to 2 months in the freezer.

DRAGONFRUIT SORBET

YIELD: 1 QUART

Although I consider most all of nature's creations beautiful, I am always awestruck each time I cut into a dragonfruit. These bright fuchsia fruits open to a Dalmatian inside and have a neutral flavor similar to grapes. They make one heck of a gorgeous sorbet, too! Check for ripeness by gently pressing into the fruit's thick peel. If it gives to a little pressure under the thumb, then it's ripe.

2 large dragonfruits

1 cup sugar

1 cup water

¼ teaspoon vanilla extract

- Peel the dragonfruit by cutting the top stem section off just enough to reveal the white fruit. Gently peel the fruit as you would a banana to remove the skin cleanly and easily.

- Cube the fruit and place into a food processor. Pulse until the consistency of a slushy.

- In a small saucepan over medium heat, cook the sugar and water together just until the sugar has completely dissolved, for 1 to 2 minutes.

- Transfer the pureed dragonfruit into a bowl and mix in the sugar syrup and vanilla. Chill the mixture in the freezer for 30 minutes, stir, chill for 10 more minutes, then process in an ice cream maker until it is bright white and the consistency of sorbet. This can also be made following the directions in this book, but an ice cream maker is preferred if available. Store in flexible airtight container in freezer for up to 3 months.

GINGER PEACH SHERBET

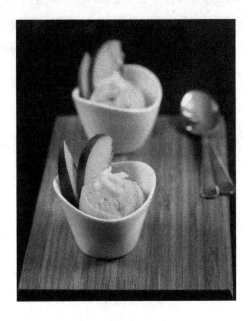

YIELD: 1 QUART

Warm ginger combines so beautifully with this cool peach sherbet to bring a dessert that would be welcome at the end of any dinner party.

4 large ripe peaches (not too soft)

1 teaspoon fresh grated ginger

Dash salt

1 cup sugar

½ cup canned full-fat coconut cream (thickest part from a can of milk)

½ cup non dairy milk

- Fill a 2-quart pot about halfway with water and bring to a boil over medium-high heat. Carefully place peaches into the boiling water and cook for 1½ minutes. Drain immediately and gently run the peaches under cold water. Carefully remove the skins and pits and discard.

- Place the blanched peaches, ginger, salt, sugar, coconut cream, and nondairy milk into a food processor or blender and blend until smooth. Chill in the refrigerator until cold and then transfer to an ice cream maker and process according to manufacturer's instructions, or follow the directions in this book. Transfer to a flexible airtight freezable container and freeze for at least 4 hours before serving. Keeps for up to 3 months frozen.

STRAWBERRY BALSAMIC SORBETTO

YIELD: 2 CUPS

An absolutely delightful dessert, this tastes just like fresh-picked strawberries. The balsamic complements the berries well and counteracts the sweetness of the simple syrup.

¾ cup <u>Simple Syrup</u>

1 tablespoon white or red balsamic vinegar

2 cups fresh strawberries, greens removed

- In a blender, puree all the ingredients until smooth. Place in metal baking dish, about 8 inches round, and cover with plastic wrap. Freeze for 3 hours, or until solid, but still soft. Store in airtight container in freezer for up to 2 months.

LIMONCELLO SEMIFREDDO

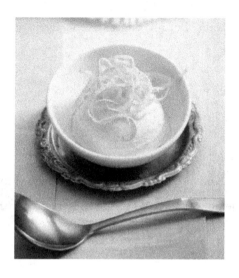

YIELD: 6 SERVINGS

A bright and boozy treat that's for adults only. This creamy, fluffy, semifreddo is best made in a high-speed blender, such as a Vitamix, for extra airiness.

2 cups raw cashews

½ cup sugar

1 cup coconut cream (from the tops of 2 chilled cans of full-fat coconut milk)

⅔ cup Limoncello

Fresh lemon zest, for garnish (optional)

- Place the cashews into a medium bowl and cover with water. Let the cashews soak for least 4 hours, but no longer than 6. Drain and place into a high-speed blender.

- Add the rest of the ingredients and blend on low just to combine. Increase speed to high and let blend until completely smooth, for about 1 minute.

- Pour the mixture into silicone baking cups or ice cream molds and freeze for at least 6 hours and up to overnight. For an extra-special touch, serve garnished with lemon zest. Keeps for up to 3 months frozen.

ALMOND CHAMOMILE GRANITA

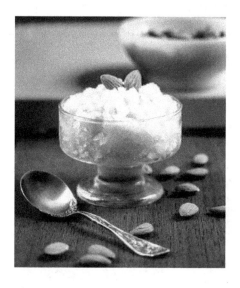

YIELD: ABOUT 3 CUPS

Such a soothing treat for a hot summer day, this light-tasting granita is a great choice when ice cream seems too heavy. The chamomile adds a floral note that's perfectly offset with the almond milk.

2 chamomile tea bags (or 2 teaspoons chamomile tea in tea strainer)

1 cup very hot, but not boiling, water

½ cup <u>Simple Syrup</u>

1 teaspoon almond extract

½ cup almond milk

* In a medium bowl, steep the tea and the hot water for 5 minutes, until the

21

water is fragrant and golden. Remove tea bags and let cool to room temperature. Mix with the syrup, almond extract, and almond milk. Place in metal baking dish, about 8 × 8 inches, on flat surface in freezer. Chill mixture until frozen solid and then scrape into granules using a fork. Serve in chilled dishes. Keeps for up to 3 months frozen if stored in airtight container.

MOJITO GRANITA

YIELD: 3 CUPS

I love mojitos in the summertime. I get giddy when I see the fresh mint peek over our fence in the springtime, letting me know it's almost time to stock up on lime and seltzer. This granita will satisfy your craving for the summertime libation any time of year.

¾ cup <u>Simple Syrup</u>

Juice of 3 limes, about 6 tablespoons

2 tablespoons rum

1 cup cold sparkling water

½ teaspoon mint extract

* Combine all the ingredients in a medium bowl, and then pour into a nonstick plastic or metal dish. Freeze for 3 hours. Once frozen, gently scrape the mixture into granules using the tines of a fork. Serve with a fresh sprig of mint or a lime twist. Store in airtight container in the freezer. Keeps for up to 3 months frozen.

MANDARIN ICE

YIELD: 1 QUART

This delightful frozen treat is a refreshing way to get your vitamin C! I like using clementines, for extra sweetness, but tangerines or other oranges work nicely, too.

1½ cups mandarin juice, about 8 clementines' worth

2 teaspoons rum or vanilla extract

1 tablespoon agave

- Place all the ingredients into a bowl and whisk together well to combine. Pour into a metal cake pan (about 9 inches round) and place into the freezer. Freeze for 4 hours, or until frozen solid. Gently but quickly scrape the mixture into ice with a fork—don't overdo it or it may turn to a slushy— and then transfer into a sealable airtight container. Keeps for up to 3 months frozen.

PINEAPPLE ICE POPS

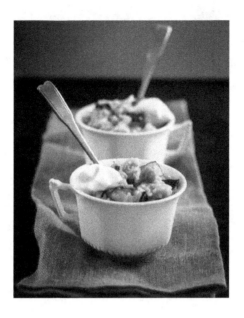

YIELD: ABOUT 4 POPS

These tropical treats are actually quite popular in Mexico and are referred to as *paleta de pina*. Paleta have countless flavor variations, but I love these pineapple pops because of the natural candy-like flavor of the pineapple.

You'll need popsicle molds or silicone ice cube trays for mini-pops or simply use small paper cups.

2 cups diced pineapple, drained

½ cup Simple Syrup

½ teaspoon rum or vanilla extract

2 tablespoons full-fat coconut milk

- Place all ingredients into a blender or food processor and blend until mostly pureed. Pour into popsicle molds, place wooden sticks into the center, and freeze overnight. Keeps for up to 3 months frozen.

Use agave in place of the simple syrup if desired, but expect a darker color to your pops.

TEMPTING PUDDINGS, CUSTARDS, JELLIES, AND FRUITS

This chapter covers everything you need to know for perfect puddings, fillings, fruits, and more. These are some of my favorite desserts to make because of the quickness and ease, as well as their uses in other desserts as fillings, toppings, and garnishes.

PUDDINGS AND CUSTARDS

CRÈME BRÛLÉE

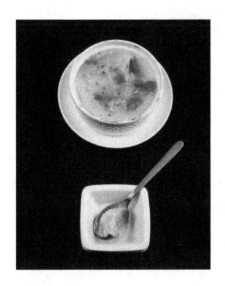

YIELD: 4 SERVINGS

If you thought that getting just the right texture for classic crème brûlée would be impossible without eggs and cream, this recipe will prove just the opposite! If you don't have a culinary torch (why not?! … they're so much fun), then you can also place these under a broiler set on high for 5 minutes; just watch carefully so that you don't burn the sugar tops.

1 (13.5-ounce) can full-fat coconut milk

1½ cups non dairy milk

1 cup water 1¾ cups sugar

3 tablespoons non dairy margarine

¾ cup cornstarch mixed with ½ cup water

3 tablespoons besan/chickpea flour

1 teaspoon vanilla extract

¾ teaspoon sea salt

2 tablespoons sugar for topping

- Prepare four ramekins by very lightly greasing them with coconut oil or margarine.

- In a 2-quart saucepan, combine the coconut milk, non dairy milk, water, sugar, and margarine and cook over medium heat for about 5 minutes, or until the mixture is hot.

- In a small bowl, mix together the cornstarch slurry, besan, and vanilla extract until very smooth. Add the cornstarch mixture into the coconut milk mixture along with the salt and stir constantly with a whisk over medium heat to let it thicken, which should happen after about 5 minutes.

- Transfer to the prepared ramekins and let cool completely at room temperature until firm. Sprinkle each cup with about ½ tablespoon sugar, then brûlée the tops using a blowtorch. Store in airtight container for up to 1 week in refrigerator.

CHOCOLATE PUDDING

YIELD: 2 TO 4 SERVINGS

One of my favorite treats is chocolate pudding. I love how involved it all seems, standing over the stove, meditatively whisking away. This pudding is just as great as other Chocolate Puddings that we know and love with its thick and creamy texture and an unforgettably chocolate flavor.

½ cup cocoa powder

½ cup sugar

2 teaspoons vanilla extract

¼ teaspoon salt

1 cup non dairy milk

3 tablespoons cornstarch

3 tablespoons water

- In a 2-quart saucepan, whisk together the cocoa powder, sugar, vanilla extract, salt, and about ⅓ cup of the non dairy milk. Mix until very smooth with no lumps remaining, and then add in the additional non dairy milk.

- Warm over medium heat. In a small bowl, whisk together the cornstarch and water until no lumps remain. Stir in the cornstarch slurry and keep stirring continuously, over medium heat, until thickened, for about 5 minutes. Transfer to two medium or four small dishes and chill before serving. Store in airtight container for up to 1 week in refrigerator.

PISTACHIO PUDDING

YIELD: 2 TO 4 SERVINGS

This slightly salty and oh-so-sweet treat is easy to bring together and a sure winner for the pistachio lover in your life. I especially love this rich pudding served in small amounts as a dessert or aperitif.

1 cup roasted and salted pistachios, shelled

½ cup granulated sugar

⅓ cup non dairy milk, plus 1½ cups non dairy milk

¼ cup additional granulated sugar

5 tablespoons cornstarch

4 tablespoons water

* In a food processor, pulse the pistachios until crumbly. Add in sugar and blend until powdery—with just a few larger chunks remaining. Add the ⅓ cup nondairy milk and puree until very well combined.

* Transfer pistachio mixture to a 2-quart pot and whisk in the additional nondairy milk and sugar.

* In a small bowl, use a fork to combine the cornstarch and water until no lumps remain. Add this slurry to the pistachio mixture.

* Heat over medium heat, stirring frequently until thickened, for 5 to 7 minutes.

Pour into two to four ramekins or serving dishes and let cool completely. Serve chilled with whipped topping! Store in airtight container for up to 1 week in refrigerator.

VANILLA PLUM RICE PUDDING

YIELD: 6 SERVINGS

A fragrant take on traditional rice pudding, I like to use basmati for its gorgeous floral notes in addition to the vanilla and plum.

¾ cup basmati or long-grain rice

1½ cups cold water

3 plums, unpeeled, stone removed, and diced

3 teaspoons vanilla extract

½ teaspoon salt

1 cup non dairy milk

½ cup sugar

2 tablespoons sweet white rice flour

¼ cup water

- In a 2- or 3-quart saucepan with a tight-fitting lid, stir together the rice and the cold water. Bring to a boil over medium-high heat. Immediately reduce to a simmer and cover. Do not stir.

- Let simmer for about 20 minutes, or until rice can be fluffed easily with a fork. Increase heat to medium and stir in the plums, vanilla extract, salt, nondairy milk, and sugar. In a smaller bowl, use a fork to stir together the

36

sweet white rice flour and water. Stir the slurry into the rice mixture and cook for about 5 to 7 minutes, stirring constantly, until thick. Serve warm or cold. Store in airtight container for up to 1 week in refrigerator.

TAPIOCA PUDDING

Tapioca pudding is one of those desserts that most people either love or hate, and I truly do adore it! Having grown up with only the instant puddings, I find this homemade version is so much better. It may change your mind if you're not a fan already. Seek out tapioca pearls in the baking section of most grocery stores, or find an endless variety of shapes and colors in Asian markets.

½ cup small tapioca pearls (not instant)

1 cup canned full-fat coconut milk

2 cups non dairy milk

½ teaspoon salt

½ cup sugar

1 teaspoon vanilla

- In a 2-quart pot, whisk together all the ingredients until smooth. Over medium-high heat, bring to a boil, stirring constantly. Once boiling, reduce heat to low and simmer for 15 minutes, stirring very often, until pudding is thickened and pearls are no longer white and firm but instead clear and gelatinous.

- Place into serving dishes or a flexible airtight container and chill until completely cold. Serve cold. Store in airtight container for up to 1 week in refrigerator.

FALL HARVEST QUINOA PUDDING

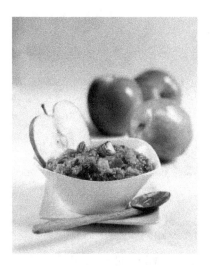

YIELD: 6 SERVINGS

Fruits and fall-time spices combine to make one comforting pudding, and the quinoa gives it a dense, creamy, and chewy texture.

1 tablespoon coconut oil

1 cup chopped pecan pieces

1 apple, chopped into small pieces

½ cup dried dates, chopped

½ teaspoon ground nutmeg

1 teaspoon ground cinnamon

¼ teaspoon cardamom

½ teaspoon salt

½ cup cold non dairy milk

2 teaspoons cornstarch

1 teaspoon vanilla extract

2 cups cooked quinoa

1 cup brown sugar

- Over medium heat, in a 2-quart saucepan, warm the coconut oil until melted. Add the pecans, apples, dates, nutmeg, cinnamon, cardamom, and salt. Continue to cook over medium heat, stirring as to not let the mixture burn. Cook for 3 to 5 minutes, or until apples soften and pecans become fragrant.

- In a small bowl, mix the non dairy milk with the cornstarch and vanilla extract. Whisk together until well combined and no lumps are visible.

- Add the cooked quinoa to the saucepan. Stir in the brown sugar and nondairy milk mixture. Cook over medium heat for about 2 minutes, or until thickened. Serve warm or chilled. Store in airtight container for up to 1 week in refrigerator.

PUMPKIN FLAN

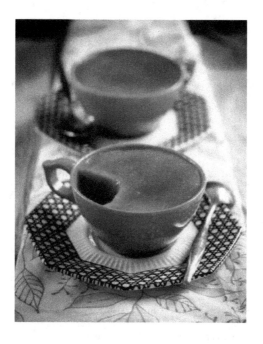

YIELD: 4 SERVINGS

This is a traditional method of making pumpkin flan, where the pumpkin is allowed to shine on its own, rather than being masked by spices like cinnamon and cloves.

1 cup canned pumpkin or strained pumpkin puree

1 cup non dairy milk

½ cup + 1 tablespoon sugar

¼ teaspoon salt

Dash ground nutmeg

⅓ cup cornstarch

4 tablespoons cold water

- Lightly grease four ramekins or teacups with margarine or cooking spray.

- In a 2-quart saucepan, whisk together the pumpkin, non dairy milk, sugar, salt, and nutmeg until smooth. Warm over medium heat.

- Combine the cornstarch with the cold water and stir until no lumps remain. Drizzle into the pumpkin mixture and continue to whisk, constantly, over medium heat until thickened, for about 7 minutes. You will notice a significant strain on your wrist as it becomes thickened.

- Pour/spoon into lightly greased ramekins and let cool. Transfer to refrigerator and chill completely until cold. Invert onto a small flat plate, or leave in cups for serving. Top with Caramel Sauce. Store in airtight container for up to 1 week in refrigerator.

CREAMSICLE CUSTARD

YIELD: 4 SERVINGS

This pudding's sunny orange flavor will brighten your day. You can even freeze this pudding in popsicle molds to make creamsicles!

4 tablespoons cornstarch

4 tablespoons cold water

2 cups non dairy milk

½ cup freshly squeezed orange juice

1 cup sugar

1 teaspoon orange zest

½ teaspoon salt

- In small bowl whisk together the cornstarch and cold water and mix well until dissolved. In a small saucepan, combine the non dairy milk, orange juice, and sugar. Stir in the zest and salt. Warm up slightly over medium- low heat, and gradually add in the cornstarch slurry while stirring frequently with a whisk until the mixture reaches a slow boil.

- Reduce heat to low and continue to stir until the mixture becomes thick, for about 10 minutes cooking time total. Divide between four serving dishes and let sit at room temperature until warm. Transfer the dishes to the refrigerator and chill for at least 3 hours, or until it is completely set. Serve chilled. Store in airtight container for up to 1 week in refrigerator.

TIRAMISU

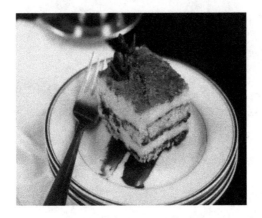

YIELD: 10 SERVINGS

Tiramisu is perhaps one of the most popular desserts at Italian restaurants. I always love Tiramisu for its intoxicating fragrance and delightfully melt-in- your-mouth texture. After going gluten-free, I was convinced this dessert would be off limits for good, but no more! Allergy-friendly fancy dessert, at your service.

10 to 12 <u>Ladyfingers</u>

¼ recipe <u>Devilishly Dark Chocolate Sauce</u>

FILLING

1 recipe <u>Mascarpone</u>

1½ cups confectioner's sugar

⅛ teaspoon salt

12 ounces firm silken tofu

3 ounces (about 3 tablespoons) non dairy cream cheese

3 tablespoons cornstarch

4 tablespoons cold water

SAUCE

1 tablespoon cocoa powder, plus more for dusting

1 tablespoon agave

2 tablespoons very strong coffee or espresso

For the Filling

- Place the Mascarpone, confectioner's sugar, salt, tofu, and nondairy cream cheese into a food processor and blend until very smooth, for about 2 minutes. Transfer the mixture into a 2-quart saucepan over medium heat.

- Whisk together the cornstarch and cold water until no lumps remain. Drizzle the cornstarch slurry into the rest of the ingredients and whisk together, continuing to cook over medium heat. Keep stirring continuously until the mixture thickens, for about 5 minutes. Do not walk away from the mixture or it will burn!

- Let cool briefly.

For the Sauce

- Prepare the sauce by whisking together the cocoa powder, agave, and coffee in a small bowl until smooth. **To assemble the Tiramisu**

- In a small, square baking pan, arrange five or six ladyfinger cookies to fit into the pan. Spread the Cocoa Espresso Sauce into a shallow flat dish, big enough for the cookies to lay flat. One by one, dip each side of the cookie into the sauce, briefly, and carefully replace. Repeat until all the cookies have been lightly dipped.

- Divide the Tiramisu filling in half and spread half of the filling on top of the ladyfingers and repeat with one more layer of each. Dust the top with cocoa powder and then drizzle with the Devilishy Dark Chocolate Sauce right before serving. Store in airtight container for up to 3 days in refrigerator.

BROWNIE BATTER MOUSSE

YIELD: 6 SERVINGS

Tiny bites of chocolate-covered walnuts—that taste a heck of a lot like miniature brownies—speckle this silky mousse, delivering a double dose of chocolate flavor.

6 ounces chopped semi-sweet chocolate

2 tablespoons non dairy milk

1 tablespoon maple syrup

1 cup roughly chopped walnuts

2 (350 g) packages extra-firm silken tofu

1 cup sugar

¾ cup cocoa powder

½ teaspoon salt

1 teaspoon vanilla extract

- Melt the chocolate in a double boiler over low heat until smooth. Stir in the nondairy milk and maple syrup and remove from the heat. Add the walnuts and coat liberally with a thick chocolate layer.

- Line a cookie sheet with a silicone mat or waxed paper. Spread the chocolate-covered walnuts in an even layer on the prepared cookie sheet. Chill the walnuts in your freezer until you are finished making the mousse.

- To make the mousse, simply blend the tofu, sugar, cocoa powder, salt, and vanilla extract in a food processor or blender until extremely smooth, for about 2 minutes, scraping down the sides as needed.

- Remove the chocolate-covered walnuts from the freezer when they are firm and stir them into the mousse. Spoon into individual dishes and serve very cold. Store in airtight container for up to 1 week in refrigerator.

BUTTERNUT POTS DE CRÈME

YIELD: 2 SERVINGS

Tender butternut squash is the base for this incredibly rich chocolate dessert. This makes a fabulous fall-time indulgence. The Pots de Crème can be made up to two days in advance.

2 cups cubed, roasted butternut squash

½ cup coconut sugar or packed brown sugar

¼ cup cocoa powder

¼ cup sorghum flour

1 teaspoon vanilla extract

½ teaspoon salt

Smoked salt for topping

- Preheat oven to 350°F and lightly grease two 4-inch ramekins.

- Puree the squash in food processor until smooth. Add in the sugar, cocoa powder, sorghum flour, vanilla extract, and salt. Blend until all ingredients are well combined, scraping the sides as needed.

- Spoon the mixture into the two ramekins and sprinkle smoked salt onto the custards. Bake for 45 to 50 minutes, or until the sides of the pudding begin to pull away from the ramekins. Serve hot for a softer pudding or serve chilled for a firm dessert. Store in airtight container for up to 1 week in refrigerator.

CHOCOLATE SOUP

YIELD: 4 SERVINGS

Somewhere in between pudding and chocolate sauce, this unusual dessert is such a fun choice for dinner parties. Serve this extra-rich dish in very small bowls.

1 cup canned coconut milk, lite or full-fat

¾ cup non dairy milk (unsweetened)

2 teaspoons vanilla extract

⅓ cup sugar

⅛ teaspoon salt

1 tablespoon cocoa powder

½ cup non dairy chocolate, chopped

1 tablespoon cornstarch mixed with 2 tablespoons water

* In a small saucepan, whisk together the coconut milk, non dairy milk, vanilla extract, sugar, salt, and cocoa powder. Heat over medium heat until very hot, but not yet boiling, for about 5 minutes. Stir in the chocolate, and heat just until melted, stirring continuously, making sure not to let the mixture come to a boil. Whisk in the cornstarch slurry and heat for about 3 minutes, stirring constantly, until the mixture has thickened and it coats the back of a spoon. Serve hot in individual bowls garnished with vegan marshmallows or Sweetened Whipped Coconut Cream and cacao nibs (or mini chocolate chips). Store in airtight container for up to 2 days in refrigerator. Reheat

simply by warming over medium-low heat in small saucepan until desired temperature is reached.

JELLIES, FRUITS, AND SAUCES

BELLINI GELEE

YIELD: 4 SERVINGS

This boozy dessert has all the crisp sweet flavor of the adult drink! Agar is used as a gelatin substitute in this gelled dessert. Be sure to dissolve the powder all the way or it won't set correctly.

1 cup peaches, blanched and pureed, or 1 cup peach nectar

1 cup sugar

3 cups Prosecco or Pinot Grigio

1 cup water

4 teaspoons agar powder

- Gather four sturdy wine glasses or medium silicone molds.

- Whisk together the pureed peaches, sugar, Prosecco, water, and agar in a 2- or 3-quart heavy saucepan. Bring to a boil, and then immediately reduce heat to low. Stir regularly and let simmer for 5 to 6 minutes.

- Let cool slightly, for about 10 minutes, before pouring into wine or champagne glasses or silicone molds.

- If you are using the silicone mold, be sure to place a larger, sturdier pan underneath the mold before you pour your liquid in, ensuring a smooth transport to the fridge.

- Let the mixture chill in the refrigerator until firm, for at least 2 hours. Store in airtight container for up to 1 week in refrigerator.

CRANBERRY FAUX-GURT

YIELD: 2 SERVINGS

The tart cranberries give this delectable treat an authentic yogurt flavor without the waiting. Top with fresh fruit and granola for an irresistible treat.

1 cup fresh cranberries

½ cup sugar or agave

1 tablespoon water

1 cup <u>Sweet Cashew Cream</u>

½ cup coconut cream (from the top of a can of coconut milk)

* In a small saucepan, over medium-low heat, cook the cranberries, sugar, and water until cranberries are very soft, for about 10 minutes. Let cool briefly and then blend in a blender along with the cashew cream and coconut cream until fluffy. Pour into jar and chill; mixture will thicken slightly upon chilling. Store in airtight container for up to 1 week in refrigerator.

CARAMEL ROASTED PEARS

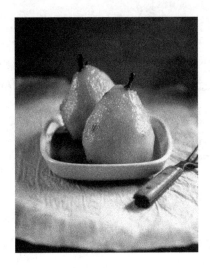

YIELD: 4 SERVINGS

This is a simple recipe, but full of complex flavor.

4 red pears, peeled but stems left intact

⅓ cup agave

⅓ cup brown sugar or coconut sugar

2 tablespoons non dairy margarine, melted

⅓ cup canned coconut milk

- Preheat oven to 400°F. Carefully slice the bottoms of the pears straight across just to remove the nodule on the bottom, so that they easily stand in a small stoneware or metal baking dish.

- In a small bowl, mix together the agave, brown sugar, margarine, and coconut milk. Drizzle generously over the pears, and then allow the rest to fall to the bottom of baking dish. Bake in a preheated oven for 25 to 30 minutes, stopping to baste with the caramel sauce every 5 minutes or so, until the pears are tender and lightly golden brown.

- Carefully transfer using a flat metal spatula to a saucer or lipped dish with the sauce drizzled onto the pears. Serve immediately. Store leftovers in an airtight container in the refrigerator for up to 2 days.

THAI MANGO STICKY RICE

YIELD: 2 SERVINGS

One of my favorite parts about visiting a Thai restaurant is enjoying the Mango Sticky Rice when mangoes are in season. Luckily, this addictive treat can be made at home! When making this recipe, it's important to seek out "glutinous" rice, usually sold as "short grain" or "sticky" rice, which refers to the glue-like stickiness of the rice, not gluten.

1 cup short-grain glutinous rice

1½ cups canned full-fat coconut milk

1 cup water

3 tablespoons sugar

Dash salt

1 mango, peeled and sliced into strips

SAUCE

½ cup canned full-fat coconut milk

1½ tablespoons sugar

1 teaspoon cornstarch

2 teaspoons water

Dash salt

- Soak 1 cup rice in 3 cups of water for 1 hour. Drain and rinse the rice and place into a saucepan with a tight-fitting lid. Stir in coconut milk, water, sugar, and salt, and bring to a boil over medium-high heat. Once it hits a boil, immediately reduce the temperature to low, stir, cover, and simmer for about 20 minutes, or until all liquid is absorbed and rice is tender.

- To make the sauce, in a small saucepan, combine the coconut milk with the sugar. In a small bowl, whisk together the cornstarch and water until smooth. Whisk the cornstarch slurry and the salt into the coconut milk mixture and cook over medium heat, stirring constantly, until thickened.

- Plate by placing a small mound of cooked rice in a bowl, along with the sliced mangos, and top with the coconut sauce. Serve immediately.

CHOICE CHOCOLATES AND DANDY CANDIES

Any candy craving can easily be satisfied at home once you get the knack for candy making—all it takes is a little patience and practice for results that far surpass store-bought. Plus, you can customize it! I've been making candy since I was tall enough to use the stove; so if you've never made candy before, don't be intimidated—even a child can do it! In this chapter you'll find recipes for everything from hard candies to chocolate treats to gooey chewy caramels.

CANDY MAKING BASICS

The best piece of advice I can give for making candy is to have all ingredients out and ready to go before beginning, and make sure you read the candy recipe instructions at least three times before beginning, until you have a clear grasp of how the recipe will work. The tricky thing about candy making is that it all happens so quickly once the sugar comes to the correct temperature, so you need to be prepared!

In the following recipes, be sure to follow the steps precisely. I recommend a (calibrated) candy thermometer for recipes requiring one, but, if you don't have one, you can always use the Cold Water Method. This is actually how I learned to make candy, so again, a very easy method that just takes a little practice to master.

COLD WATER METHOD

Place cup of ice-cold water next to your saucepan containing your candy mixture. Test for the candy doneness by dropping about a teaspoon or so of the hot syrup from a spoon into the cold water. Follow the temperature guidelines below, which outline the properties of the candy at each stage of doneness

Soft-Ball Stage

235°F–240°F

A soft, flexible ball that will flatten when removed from water.

Firm-Ball Stage

245°F–250°F

A firm ball that will hold its shape when removed from the water but is malleable.

Hard-Ball Stage

250°F–265°F

A firm ball that is a little more difficult to change the shape, but possible.

Soft-Crack Stage

270°F–290°F

Flexible threads will form when dropped into ice-cold water.

Hard-Crack Stage

300°F–310°F

This is the hottest stage of most candy recipes, so be sure to let the dropped syrup cool completely in the water before touching it in this stage. When sugar is dropped into the cold water, brittle hard threads will form.

WASH DOWN

When cooking sugar into candy, be sure to wash down the sugar crystals from the sides of the pan as you go. You can do this simply with a silicone brush dipped in a running stream of water. Just brush lightly over the crystals, as many times as needed, until all crystals are dissolved. This is important as a single sugar crystal can cause recrystallization, ruining the whole batch of candy. Always have a silicone or bristle brush handy to wash down the sides of your saucepan.

__SAUCEPAN__

When making candy it is important that you use a good-quality saucepan for best heat distribution. Too thin of a saucepan can cause scorching and other unpleasantries. You don't need to spend a lot of money, though; one of my favorite candy-making pots is an old Revere Ware copper-bottomed 3-quart pan that I learned to make candy with as a kid. It still serves me well today. I recommend a 2- or 3-quart pan for all the recipes listed, unless otherwise specified. Also, make sure that the sides of the pan are straight, so that you can get an accurate read on your thermometer.

CHOOSING QUALITY CHOCOLATE

When you're out perusing the specialty food stores or hobby shops, you may notice that there are basically two different types of chocolate to choose from: couverture and baking chips, such as Ghirardelli. Couverture is very high quality chocolate that contains extra cocoa butter. You may be unable to find good-quality couverture at a supermarket but seek it out at specialty groceries, craft stores, or even online. Amazon has a good selection of dairy-free couverture at excellent prices.

The main difference between couverture and baking chips is the final outcome of the chocolate. Couverture results in a snappy, shiny texture (like chocolates from chocolatiers and patisseries), and chocolate chips—when used to coat—oftentimes have a softer texture that's best if kept chilled in the refrigerator. And, it's never shiny. There are benefits to using both, and I'll let you decide what type of chocolate you choose when making chocolates and other confections. But, quality counts, so regardless of whether or not you decide to temper, be sure to seek out the best-tasting, highest-quality chocolate you can afford when chocolate making (we'll talk about tempering below).

For couverture, most chocolate over 55 percent is dairy-free, making it suitable for vegans. I like Guittard and Barry-Callebaut brands. Coppeneur Germany is a great brand for soy-free.

TEMPERING CHOCOLATE 101

While it is simple to coat candies and other confections in melted chocolate chips, resulting in an even, soft layer of chocolate, tempering is the process that gives hardened chocolate the typical snap and shine of professional chocolates. Tempering chocolate may seem daunting, especially if you've never even heard of it, but I assure you, just like anything, with a little practice, you'll soon have perfect results. You must gather a few required ingredients and tools before attempting to temper chocolate:

1. High-quality couverture chocolate

2. A double boiler/bain marie or stainless steel bowl and saucepan to act as a double boiler

3. A chocolate thermometer. Be sure to seek out a thermometer made for chocolate, or one that reaches a temperature of at least 80°F accurately and measures in small increments.

4. Patience and persistence

5. Chocolate molds (and chocolate gloves)

When you first begin tempering, you may feel nervous; rest assured, you can always let the chocolate cool and then start all over again if you've messed up. Plus, once you finally nail tempering, you will have a remarkable sense of satisfaction. The gorgeous sheen and tight snap from tempered chocolate is well worth the additional effort, which is mostly wait time.

To temper, follow these instructions, making sure never to allow any water near or around the chocolate. If water hits the chocolate, it will be ruined—even the teensiest amount—and you won't be able to ever temper it. I also recommend using a stainless steel bowl to temper rather than stoneware or glass, as the latter tends to retain heat longer, which can be problematic for tempering.

Also, keep in mind that different couverture brands and percentages of cocoa can and will have different tempering temperatures. The directions below outline a general guideline for dark chocolate, about 61 to 66 percent cocoa content.

1. Over medium-low heat, warm about 1 to 2 inches of water in a double boiler. Place the required amount of couverture (chopped or in coins, don't grate it) into the bowl of the double boiler while the water is still cool, making sure not to get any water whatsoever on the couverture. Melt the chocolate completely, stirring occasionally and heat to 115–120°F. Remove from heat and let cool to about 82°F, stirring occasionally. Once at that temperature, drop about 1 teaspoon of already tempered solid chocolate (about 3 coins from the bag of chocolate you are using) into the melted couverture. Stir a lot. This is called "seeding."

2. Place the double boiler bowl back onto medium-low and heat while stirring, until the temperature of the chocolate is increased to 88– 91°F; once in this range, remove from heat. Do not let it get above 91°F or it won't temper. Keep a close eye on the chocolate during this step as it reheats quickly.

3. Voilà! You have tempered chocolate. If there is any remaining "seed" chocolate, remove it before dipping, coating, or molding. Once your chocolate is tempered it should set quickly (about 20 minutes) at room temperature and will appear shiny and "snappy" when bitten into. Use in

molds or to coat candies, such as the Buttery Fingers or to coat the Salted Espresso Truffles. Don't place the chocolate in the refrigerator, or it will cause "bloom," which is white streaks in chocolate that form from cocoa butter separating.

CLASSIC CANDIES

LOLLIPOPS OR HARD CANDY

YIELD: 20 CANDIES

Have you ever thought to make your own lollipops? If not, now's the time! They are easy as can be and you can completely control the flavor. One trip to a craft or candy supply store and you'll have what it takes to make enough lollies to last a year! Seek out white plastic molds as they are made specifically for molding hard candies and releasing without breakage.

1 cup sugar

½ cup water

⅛ teaspoon cream of tartar

1 to 2 drops food coloring (optional)

½ teaspoon flavored oil or extract, such as lemon or cherry

- Place the plastic (white) hard candy molds onto a flat surface and place in the lollipop sticks, if you're using them. Have the molds nearby for when your sugar is ready to go.

- Over medium heat, in a 2- or 3-quart saucepan, combine the sugar, water, and cream of tartar and heat until boiling, stirring often as it cooks. Be sure to brush down the sides of the pan with a wet pastry brush once the sugar crystals mostly are dissolved. Once the mixture is boiling, stop stirring.

- Clip on a candy thermometer. Let mixture cook until the candy thermometer reaches 300°F (or Hard Crack Stage using the Cold Water Method) or until it turns from clear to a very light caramel hue.

- Working quickly, immediately stir the food coloring and flavoring into the pot. Pour the mixture into candy molds. Rap the mold lightly on flat surface to remove any air bubbles from the candy, and let the candies set until totally hardened. Pop out and place onto waxed paper. Store in airtight container for up to 1 month.

Silicone molds are the best to use, in my opinion, when making hard candies. But, white plastic molds can be used, too. I find the plastic lollipop molds release easiest when candy is still very warm, but firm.

ENGLISH TOFFEE

YIELD: 8 SERVINGS

This crunchy toffee is coated with decadent dark chocolate and topped with toasted nuts. If you have a nut allergy, replace with toasted sunflower or hemp seeds, which will be just as delicious, or leave them off altogether. In the unlikely event you find yourself with leftover candy, this recipe makes a fabulous mix-in to ice cream when crushed and stirred in after the ice cream has churned. Or, try it instead of chocolate chips in the Classic Chocolate Chip Cookies.

1½ cups non dairy margarine

1½ cups sugar

¼ teaspoon salt

2 cups non dairy chocolate chips

1 cup nuts (such as almonds or pecans), toasted and chopped

Prepare a cookie sheet or jelly roll pan with enough parchment paper or a silicone mat to cover.

* Combine the margarine, sugar, and salt in a 2-quart saucepan and melt gently over medium heat, stirring often.

* Continue stirring as the mixture hits a boil, and keep cooking until the candy mixture reaches 300°F on your candy thermometer (for about 30 minutes or Hard Crack Stage if you're using the Cold Water Method). Immediately pour liquid candy mixture onto the prepared surface and spread until about ¼ inch thick. Let cool for about 3 minutes, or until slightly firm, and then carefully

place the chocolate chips into an even layer on top of the hot toffee. Allow the chips to rest for about 2 minutes, and then use a silicone spatula to smooth the chocolate over the top of the toffee.

- Sprinkle with nuts and allow to cool completely. Break into bite-size pieces. Store in airtight container for up to 1 month.

BUTTERY FINGERS

YIELD: 8 SERVINGS

These irresistible candies taste just like the commercial brand, with addictively crunchy peanut butter candy layers encased in creamy chocolate. Of course, these are just as nice without the chocolate on the outside … especially when crumbled up and sprinkled on ice cream.

1 cup sugar

⅓ cup corn syrup

⅓ cup water, room temperature

1 cup creamy peanut butter

1 teaspoon vanilla extract

2 cups couverture, tempered (see recipe)

- Line a 9 × 13-inch baking sheet with parchment paper or have ready a silicone baking mat the same size.

- In a 2-quart saucepan combine the sugar, corn syrup, and water. Bring to a boil over medium heat, stirring often with a clean wooden spoon and washing down sides with a silicone brush. Once boiling, reduce stirring to occasionally until mixture reads 290°F on a candy thermometer (or the Soft Crack Stage if using the Cold Water Method).

- Remove from heat immediately and quickly stir in the peanut butter and vanilla extract and spread about ½ inch thick onto the baking sheet or silicone baking mat. Score lightly using a sharp knife and break into 1 × 2 inch-bars.

- Cover with tempered couverture and let the candy set until the chocolate becomes firm, for about 1 to 2 hours. Store in an airtight container for up to 1 month.

You can replace the corn syrup here with agave to make it corn-free, although the color of the candy will be darker and it may have a slightly different taste than traditional Butter-finger candy.

ALLERGY NOTE

For a corn-free version, use agave rather than corn syrup.

CANDY KETTLE CORN

YIELD: 5½ CUPS

Such a fun treat to serve at Halloween, or anytime! The sweet and salty combo of kettle corn is hard to resist, so be sure to double the recipe if making for a large crowd.

5½ cups popped popcorn, salted to taste (about ½ cup unpopped kernels)

2 cups sugar

1 cup light corn syrup or agave

½ cup non dairy margarine

¼ cup apple cider

1 teaspoon vanilla extract

1 teaspoon apple cider vinegar

1 cup non dairy chocolate chips

⅔ cup sliced almonds, toasted

- Make sure your popcorn is popped and set aside, ready to go in a large bowl. Have nearby a candy thermometer and a wooden spoon.

- Grease a 9 × 13-inch cookie sheet.

- In a heavy saucepan, at least 8 inches deep, combine the sugar, corn syrup, margarine, and apple cider. Over medium heat, bring the mixture to boil, stirring occasionally. Continue to cook over medium heat and stir regularly using a wooden spoon until your candy thermometer reads 300°F (or Hard

Crack Stage if using the Cold Water Method). This takes a while. Patience totally pays off with these, so don't rush and pull the candy from the stove before it reaches hard crack stage. Be sure to wash down (<u>recipe</u>) the sides!

- Remove the candy mixture from the heat and quickly stir in the vanilla extract and vinegar. Pour HOT candy mixture over the popcorn and stir quickly until evenly coated. Let cool for about 5 to 7 minutes. Spread onto a greased cookie sheet and let cool completely.

- Using a double boiler, melt the chocolate until smooth. Drizzle melted chocolate over the candied popcorn and sprinkle with sliced almonds. Let chocolate harden and then break into bite-size pieces. Store in an airtight container in the fridge or a cool place where chocolate will not melt for up to 1 month.

To easily toast almonds, spread in an even layer on a cookie sheet and bake for 7 minutes at 375°F, or until fragrant.

PINWHEEL CANDY

YIELD: 20 PIECES

There is much speculation about the origins of this candy, ranging from German, to Irish, to Pennsylvania Dutch, to the product of ingenuity during the Great Depression when limited ingredients were all there were to work with, which may be why potatoes are a key ingredient here. Even though potatoes aren't normally thought of as dessert food, they really do work quite nicely in this recipe! I recommend using a Yukon Gold or similar variety; if you opt for russet, you may need a touch more nondairy milk to make smooth.

1 large medium-to low-starch potato, peeled, mashed, and salted lightly

¼ cup non dairy milk

1 teaspoon vanilla extract

½ teaspoon salt

2 pounds (about 6 cups) confectioners sugar (or enough to make stiff dough)

About 1 cup chocolate hazelnut butter (such as Justin's brand)

- In a large bowl, combine the mashed potatoes, non dairy milk, vanilla extract, and sea salt until smooth. Gradually incorporate the confectioner's sugar until a stiff dough forms. You may need a little more or a little less sugar depending on the moisture level of your mashed potatoes.

- Form the dough into a large patty and refrigerate for at least 2 hours. Place the chilled dough in between two sheets of plastic wrap and roll out into a rectangle about ½ inch thick. Slather generously with chocolate hazelnut butter until coated. Using the bottom piece of the plastic wrap, gently guide the dough into a roll longways as you would a jelly roll. Cover with plastic wrap and chill for an additional hour. Once chilled, cut into ½-inch-wide sections and wrap in waxed paper, twisting each side to close.

* Store in fridge in airtight container. Keeps for up to 1 week.

AFTER DINNER MINTS

YIELD: 80 MINTS

These mints are easy to whip up but impressive enough to brag about when serving to friends. Call them artisan and watch their eyes light up.

Note that you can feel free to sub in Sweet Cashew Cream for the cream cheese, just add a little more confectioner's sugar until it reaches the correct consistency.

8 ounces nondairy cream cheese

1 tablespoon non dairy margarine

2 drops pure peppermint extract/oil

Food coloring paste (use corn-free if needed)

3½ to 4 cups confectioner's sugar, plus extra for dusting (use corn-free if needed)

- Mix the cream cheese, margarine, peppermint oil, and food coloring with a whisk until smooth. Gradually add in the confectioner's sugar, about ½ cup at a time, until a stiff dough forms—much like Play-Doh.

- Pat into a disk and roll out in between two sheets of parchment paper. Cut with a very small cookie cutter (or use a knife/pizza cutter to cut into squares) into desired shapes and then place on cookie tray that will fit in your fridge. Chill for 1 hour, then transfer to a resealable plastic container to store for up to 1 month in refrigerator. These also freeze well and can be thawed in your refrigerator until eating.

MARZIPAN

YIELD: 10 SERVINGS

Sold in tiny tubes at specialty stores or in the baking aisle of your neighborhood grocery, marzipan is easy to make at home, saving you both money and the effort of finding one that is dairy-, egg- and gluten-free, which can be difficult. Bonus: almonds, the main ingredient here, are tiny powerhouses rich in calcium, iron, potassium, magnesium, copper, and zinc!

1 tablespoon flaxseed meal

2 tablespoons water

3 cups blanched almond meal

1 cup confectioners sugar, plus extra for rolling

Dash salt

- In a small bowl, combine the flaxseed meal with the water and allow to rest until thickened, for about 5 minutes.

- In a food processor, blend the 3 cups almond meal until clumpy and the texture becomes somewhat like a paste, scraping down the sides and bottom of the bowl often. It should take 7 to 10 minutes' blending time to become clumpy.

- Add the confectioner's sugar and salt and pulse until once again crumbly, for about 30 seconds to 1 minute. Drizzle in about half of the prepared flaxseed meal while the food processor is blending and continue to add a little more until the mixture clumps together into a dough. Remove from food processor and form into a cylinder. Roll out gently onto a confectioner's sugar–covered surface and then wrap tightly to store. Use immediately or keep refrigerated for up to 2 weeks.

SIMPLE WHITE CHOCOLATE

YIELD: 8 OUNCES

This confection is best used for baking or candy making, rather than straight snacking, but it's perfect for the recipes in this book that call for white chocolate. Seek out the highest-quality food-grade cacao butter you can find for top-quality flavor.

8 ounces food-grade cacao butter, chopped into ½-inch pieces

¼ cup soy milk powder

3 tablespoons agave

⅓ cup confectioners sugar

⅛ teaspoon salt

1 teaspoon vanilla extract

• In a double boiler, over medium-low heat, melt the cacao butter until completely liquefied. Whisk in the soymilk powder until completely dissolved. Stir in the agave, confectioner's sugar, salt, and vanilla extract and whisk again until very well blended with no lumps remaining. Pour straight into a plastic or silicone chocolate mold and refrigerate for 20 minutes until solid. Pop out of mold and use as desired. Store in airtight container for up to 1 month.

CHOCOLATE ALMOND NUGGETS

YIELD: 10 SERVINGS

As a child, one of my favorite candy combinations was simply chocolate with almonds. These bite-size morsels are a tribute to these two "made for each other" flavors.

½ cup sliced almonds

1 cup non dairy chocolate

¼ cup almond meal

- Preheat oven to 375°F and spread the almonds onto a baking tray. Bake for 7 minutes, or until fragrant. Watch carefully so that they do not burn.

- Melt chocolate over a double boiler until totally smooth. Stir in the almond meal and toasted almonds. Drop by small spoonfuls onto waxed paper or a silicone mat. Let harden completely. Store in airtight container for up to 3 weeks.

METRIC CONVERSIONS

The recipes in this book have not been tested with metric measurements, so some variations might occur.

Remember that the weight of dry ingredients varies according to the volume or density factor: 1 cup of flour weighs far less than 1 cup of sugar, and 1 tablespoon doesn't necessarily hold 3 teaspoons.

General Formula for Metric Conversion

Ounces to grams   multiply ounces by 28.35

Grams to ounces   multiply ounces by 0.035

Pounds to grams   multiply pounds by 453.5

Pounds to kilograms   multiply pounds by 0.45

Cups to liters   multiply cups by 0.24

Fahrenheit to Celsius   subtract 32 from Fahrenheit

temperature, multiply by 5, divide by 9

Celsius to Fahrenheit   multiply Celsius temperature by 9,

divide by 5, add 32

Volume (Liquid) Measurements

1 teaspoon = ⅙ fluid ounce = 5 milliliters

1 tablespoon = ½ fluid ounce = 15 milliliters 2 tablespoons = 1 fluid ounce = 30 milliliters

¼ cup = 2 fluid ounces = 60 milliliters

⅓ cup = 2⅔ fluid ounces = 79 milliliters

½ cup = 4 fluid ounces = 118 milliliters

1 cup or ½ pint = 8 fluid ounces = 250 milliliters

2 cups or 1 pint = 16 fluid ounces = 500 milliliters

4 cups or 1 quart = 32 fluid ounces = 1,000 milliliters

1 gallon = 4 liters

Oven Temperature Equivalents, Fahrenheit (F) and Celsius (C)

100°F = 38°C

200°F = 95°C

250°F = 120°C

300°F = 150°C

350°F = 180°C

400°F = 205°C

450°F = 230°C

Volume (Dry) Measurements

¼ teaspoon = 1 milliliter

½ teaspoon = 2 milliliters

¾ teaspoon = 4 milliliters 1 teaspoon = 5 milliliters

1 tablespoon = 15 milliliters

¼ cup = 59 milliliters

⅓ cup = 79 milliliters

½ cup = 118 milliliters

⅔ cup = 158 milliliters

¾ cup = 177 milliliters 1 cup = 225 milliliters

4 cups or 1 quart = 1 liter

½ gallon = 2 liters 1 gallon = 4 liters

Linear Measurements

½ in = 1½ cm

1 inch = 2½ cm

6 inches = 15 cm

8 inches = 20 cm

10 inches = 25 cm

12 inches = 30 cm

20 inches = 50 cm